FINDING PEACE & HOPE IN THE STORM:
A CHRISTIAN WOMAN'S INFERTILITY JOURNEY

Talisha A. Matheson

Copyright © 2024 by The Inspired Introvert/Talisha A Matheson

ISBN: 978-1-7777453-6-3

All rights reserved.

No part of this publication may be reproduced,
stored in a retrieval system or transmitted in any form or by
any means – electronic, mechanical, photocopying, recording
or otherwise – without prior written permission from the author.

Disclaimer/Trigger Warning:

This book contains sensitive and potentially distressing content related to infertility, including emotional struggles and medical procedures; therefore, reader discretion is advised.

The journey depicted in this book is a profoundly personal account of my own experiences with infertility. Every story, emotion, and reflection within these pages belongs to me and is recounted in my words. While this narrative aims to offer insight, support, and empathy to those navigating similar challenges, it is essential to recognize that each individual's journey through infertility is unique.

This book does not intend to provide medical advice or professional or spiritual counselling.

Readers are encouraged to seek appropriate guidance and support from qualified healthcare professionals and support networks.

INTRODUCTION

I suppose being at a loss for words on the opening page of this book is not necessarily setting me on the right foot, but stick with me as I gather my bearings as we broach this sensitive topic together.

Infertility is a unique and profound suffering, and for many of us facing it, the initial reaction to God's apparent "no" will naturally be met with resistance and heartache. However, through prayer, reflection, and seeking guidance from scripture, rather than viewing infertility as a roadblock to our dreams, many find purpose in using their journey to uplift and support others in similar circumstances and can find solace in knowing that God's plans are far greater than our own.

While the path may be fraught with uncertainty and disappointment, may we find comfort in knowing that every trial and perceived unanswered prayer is part of a greater plan orchestrated by a magnificent, loving and sovereign God.

If we are willing to, we learn what it means to lean not on our understanding but to trust in God's perfect plan for our lives. His presence is where we find purpose, meaning, and a deeper connection to our faith. Our stories, though hard to share sometimes, will serve as a testament to the transformative power of surrendering to God's will and trusting in His unfailing love and provision.

As much as I wrote this book to help others, it has helped me tremendously. I feel as if this leg of my journey is about being open.
It's about sharing.

If you are reading this because you are on the journey, I pray you find comfort and encouragement between the lines. If you are reading this because you want to know how to support someone on this journey and don't know how, I pray this gives you some insight into navigating this trial with your loved one.

DEAR READER

Welcome to **Finding Faith & Hope in the Storm: A Christian Woman's Fertility Journey.** I would love to say this book was easy to write, but it was one of the hardest things I have ever written. It took a lot of prayer and discernment to ensure I wrote from a place of transparency and that you, my reader, saw God's grace and mercy throughout it all because I was merely a vessel despite the story being mine.

For those who know me, much of what you will read may be a shock because I went through this journey without knowing how I truly felt and how it impacted me over the years. After thinking about why I chose to do it alone, I concluded that I never felt anyone could relate to me and decided to keep it to myself.

Although I am far from the beginning, I am still on the journey and think of my infertility often. I knew I needed to do something with the trial God allowed me to go through, but I didn't know when or how it would be used until one night while reading a devotional. It was as if its author had written that day's words specifically for me. It said (I am paraphrasing) that the trials we go through are often used to help others, and keeping these stories and testimonies to ourselves is an act of disobedience.

And there it was, both convicting and encouraging, as I was directed to write and share my story of infertility as a single Christian woman and speak on how it changes how one navigates life and how, if you are a believer, it significantly alters your relationship with yourself and God.

So, in complete obedience to the nudging of the Holy Spirit, with shaking knees, a palpitating heart, and a knot in my stomach, I present this book as a testimony of finding peace and hope in the storm.

Be Blessed & Be Inspired!

**FEAR THOU NOT;
FOR I AM WITH THEE:
BE NOT DISMAYED;
FOR I AM THY GOD:
I WILL STRENGTHEN THEE;
YEA, I WILL HELP THEE;
YEA, I WILL UPHOLD THEE
WITH THE RIGHT HAND
OF MY RIGHTEOUSNESS.**

Isaiah 41:10 KJV

PROGNOSIS & DIAGNOSIS

It was March 2011; I was in the best health of my life. I had just lost a substantial amount of weight and finally hit my weight loss goal on my 32nd birthday the month prior. I finally felt comfortable in my skin. The other things going on in my life were "up in the air," to say the least, but when it came to my health and body image, it was the one thing I had under control, or at least I thought I did.

By mid-March, whenever I lay on my stomach, I felt a lump in my abdomen. When I lay on my back and touched my lower abdomen, I could still feel the lump. I convinced myself that I was merely getting used to a new body. I went for my yearly physical to showcase my weight loss to a doctor who always told me I needed to 'lose a little weight.' That day, after he congratulated me on my progress, he also discovered the lump without me needing to tell him about it. That day changed the rest of my life and strapped me into a rollercoaster that I was unprepared to be on.

My initial diagnosis was a grapefruit-sized fibroid tumour on the outside of my uterus, and my doctor told me that there was nothing to worry about, so I didn't worry. I was living my life, travelling and doing everything a woman in her early 30s does. Perhaps I was naive because I knew many women who had fibroids and also had children, and I didn't feel as if I had to be concerned with my fertility. We 'watched and waited' as my doctors recommended to see if my fibroids would shrink, stay the same or grow. And grow they did at an alarming pace my doctors were not expecting nor comfortable with.

My weight and pain increased, and I went from not requiring surgery to having an invasive procedure in early 2014 to remove what grew from a grapefruit-sized to a cantaloupe-sized fibroid on my uterus—leaving me with severely damaged abdominal nerves and a large horizontal scar across my abdomen.

Still not easily void of hope, I told myself that women are diagnosed with fibroids all the time, and once removed, that would be the end of it. Unfortunately, that was not the case.

After that surgery, my gynecologist told me there were a lot more fibroids on the inside and outside of my uterus that never revealed themselves on my numerous internal and external ultrasounds and endless MRIs. She reassured me that since they were all small, there was nothing for me to worry about. So, I went on about my life, but something still didn't feel right and worry slowly crept in.

My calendar was full for months, not with social outings but with doctor and specialist appointments. I was on a six to eight-week medical schedule, seeing my family doctor, gynecologist and fertility specialist, all while trying different drug treatments.

I distinctly remember being on one drug designed to shrink cancerous tumours in patients, and that's when I knew my condition was far more severe than my medical team was revealing. After six months and six scans, my fibroids were multiplying, and yet another drug failed at doing what the doctors were hoping they would do. I was both tired and discouraged. Prayer and laying hands on my body was something I often did, not to mention hoping I would wake up from a terrible nightmare and, most of all, that I would be well.

I remember, as if it were yesterday, after an extensive and complicated MRI, as I got dressed in the changing room, I overheard the technologists who oversaw my scan whisper among themselves that my womb was damaged. Imagine strangers having a candid conversation about a part of your body that you associated with womanhood as damaged. That encounter confirmed what I had already believed at the time: that not only was my womb damaged, but so was I.

I was mentally, physically and spiritually exhausted and as much as I wanted to have hope, it was slowly fading.

By late 2015, the pain had intensified, and other symptoms throughout my body began manifesting. My entire body was engrossed in pain. Migraines were frequent, my joints were on fire, my lower back and legs were in a constant state of ache and swelling, and no amount of stretching or medication gave me relief.

My final diagnosis was bleak, and doctors described my situation as an abdomen covered in fibroids on the inside and outside of my uterus with blocked fallopian tubes and a severe case of final staged Adenomyosis (ad-uh-no-my-O-sis).

As an aside, from what I remember from my endless hours of research, Adenomyosis is a condition that typically affects women in their 40s and 50s who have had past abortions and or pregnancies and in my mid-30s, I had neither. The condition occurs when the tissue that lines the uterus grows into its muscular wall. The abnormal tissue, while causing excruciating pain, also tricked my body into thinking I was having a regular cycle every month despite there being nothing ordinary about it. So, there I was, 36, single and medically infertile.

No matter how much I prayed for healing, I felt as if God was silent, and I had no idea how to process it all. And unfortunately, there wasn't anyone who truly understood my position. I had feelings of rejection, abandonment, loneliness, anger, physical and emotional pain and an overwhelming sense of shame. The devastating combination of my diagnosis and unfamiliar emotions led me to bury my feelings and act as if I was okay because pretending was more manageable than facing it head-on, especially when there didn't seem to be any answers.

I worked myself to exhaustion day after day, taking on special projects and additional tasks to fill my headspace and distract me from dealing with everything happening in my life. I acted as if nothing was wrong during the day and would go home in the evening and continue acting as if everything was fine. Sundays would roll around, and I would go to church, teach Sunday school, and play my violin in the orchestra with tears streaming down my face, all while acting as if everything was okay. Monday would come, and I would do it all over again.

My body felt broken, my soul was in tatters, and I felt alone, and day after day, month after month, I acted as if I wasn't coming apart at the seams. I pretended that I didn't cry myself to sleep most nights and instead covered myself in a Teflon exterior that, now, when I look back at it, was the armour that nearly destroyed me.

JESUS, I DON'T UNDERSTAND,
BUT I WILL TRUST YOU,
KNOWING YOU ALWAYS LEAD ME
IN THE BEST WAY.

AMEN

EMOTIONAL ROLLER COASTER

The thrill-seeker in me loves an exhilarating roller coaster. There is something about the adrenalin-inducing climb to the top, the pause and then the sudden drop. You feel as if your stomach will leap from your body. The quick twists and turns put you in a state of delirium, and the beauty is that you can always anticipate the next movement. It's the adrenalin rush of your life, and then, as things slow down, you come to a screeching halt and regain your senses. There is an odd satisfaction of conquering the roller coaster; if you're not too dizzy, you want to do it again. I appreciate those roller coasters. It's predictable at every turn. You know when it will begin and end, unlike the emotional ride infertility puts you on.

I lost count of the times I asked, "Why Me, God?" I am not proud that I questioned God, but in full transparency, I did so often because I wanted to know. I needed to know. I needed to understand why God would allow my womb to close yet allow the wombs of women who aborted and would abort future babies open. I needed to know why this was happening to me when I was faithful in serving him daily. I needed to understand why he was allowing this to happen and perhaps why he didn't wait until after I was married with a child or two before this terrible thing invaded my life. The biggest question of all is why he would deliver me from the grips of being aborted from my mother's womb over 30 years prior, only to allow my womb to be shut. I needed to know the answer to the age-old question, "Why, Lord, is this happening to me?"

Perhaps those reading this can relate and understand the depth and excruciating pain associated with asking the creator why your situation is plaguing your life. Maybe you are walking the tightrope of believing God for healing one day and then treading the waters of loss and despair the other. It's an exhausting battle, especially when you posture yourself in front of the Lord to pray and have no words to say. You sit with your Bible in front of you and have no idea what book or verse you need to turn to for comfort, and every memory verse you learned as a child in Sunday School escapes you at the exact time you need it.

These situations happened often, and one day, after years of suffering physically and mentally, I had no choice but to stop asking, and that is when the Lord answered my silence with a question. "Why not you?" There it was; I couldn't answer why it couldn't or shouldn't have been me, and I had to learn to stop asking and replace my questions with scripture. Isaiah 41:13 tells us: *For I the Lord thy God will hold thy right hand, saying unto thee, Fear not; I will help thee.*

After much spiritual growth, I realize that the enemy will plant seeds of doubt and will try to convince you that God does not care for you, but that is a lie from the pit of hell. God cares for you and will see you through your trial, no matter how it looks or the outcome.

We serve a gentle, loving, and sovereign God who knows us better than we know ourselves. He comforts us in all situations. He is still there when we are numb and can't feel his presence. Amid our questioning, anger, pain, and turmoil, he loves us and is close enough to hold us and remind us that He is our help. Isaiah 41:13 is bursting with hope, which I pray may encourage you to trust that God, our creator, has a reason and a plan for the trial you are going through.

SERVING GOD WHEN THE STORM IS RAGING

I'm a church girl, and attending church weekly, playing my violin in the orchestra, and teaching Sunday school was often difficult. I sang hymns but didn't believe the words half the time because they contradicted my condition. I couldn't sing "It is well with my soul" because my soul was in tatters. As we would sing about the goodness of God and praise him, I was so deep in my suffering that no matter how hard I tried to meditate on the words and have confidence in his goodness, I always felt as if God's goodness wasn't meant for me.

I was reading my Bible and doing my devotionals, and it was as if the verses were not impacting me. I would be in the middle of praise and worship and feeling God's presence, and as soon as it was over, I would return to worrying. Shame soon crept in because how could I be in the presence of God yet still feel so sad?

I am saying all of this because I want to acknowledge the difficulty of living with fertility issues while being a woman of faith, as it adds a layer to an already difficult struggle that I am not sure many understand.

I always felt as if I needed to "move past" and "get over" the anger, hopelessness, despair and lingering sadness because to have such feelings was a sign of a lack of faith, but that is the furthest from the truth. Eventually, I realized the moment I was honest with God about how I felt, especially when it came to Him, was the moment He met me where I was, forgave me and covered me continually.

SINGLE, INFERTILE & LONELY

As the youngest of three, I never entirely understood loneliness. I always had someone to play with, whether a reluctant sibling, myself or an imaginary friend. As an adult, I enjoy my own company and have no issue spending hours, days or weeks alone, so to say being alone doesn't bother me is an understatement. Loneliness, on the other hand, was a feeling I never experienced until my diagnosis, and not only did I not know what to do with such a foreign feeling, I also didn't have the words to express how I felt.

It is the Lord who goes before you.
He will be with you; he will not leave you or forsake you.
Do not fear or be dismayed.

Deuteronomy 31:8 ESV

To be forsaken is to feel abandoned or deserted, and my loneliness eventually turned into a deep feeling of being forsaken. There were times on the front end of my journey when I isolated myself to the point that God felt far away. It wasn't because he had abandoned me but because I had pushed him so far away and refused to be in his presence consistently. I was mad at him and couldn't understand why a loving God would allow me to go through this specific trial at such a critical point in my life and why he would allow me to be surrounded by people who didn't understand.

My lack of understanding during that time caused me to feel uncomfortable in his presence, and I was incapable of focusing on his goodness, which left me unable to trust Him fully. That's when loneliness crept in and enveloped me like a flood, and I couldn't swim.

Perhaps some of you are experiencing this overwhelming feeling, and you have concluded, like I have, that those who never struggled with their fertility don't understand. In contrast, others have varying levels of understanding depending on where they are on the journey or how it ended.

Some women understand the hysterectomy but don't understand the impact of infertility because they already have children. Many understand the struggle of fertility issues but don't understand childlessness. While the rest understand both, they don't quite comprehend the complex layer singleness and faith add to it.

Speaking from the perspective of a Christian, single, childless and infertile woman, I can attest to the fact that this is a lonely journey despite having people around. It is the type of loneliness where the only sound you can hear are the echoes of your weeping, and the only comfort you sometimes feel are the tears as they roll down your face. I am painting this picture because I need you to know that I understand, and for those who are reading this as a support to someone you love who is going through this trial, I need you also to have a picture of what your loved one is possibly going through.

If you are single and infertile, the enemy will try to tell you that a part of you is broken and, therefore, renders you as not enough. The enemy will tell you that you are incomplete and something is wrong with you. He will tell you that you are not worthy and that God doesn't care about you.

The enemy will attack your self-esteem from every angle to try to thwart God's plan for your life. He will tell you that no one will want you because you cannot have children. It was easy for me to believe what the enemy told me because when dating, men would change their minds about me and say the reason was because they wanted children, and I wasn't able to provide that. But then Jesus stepped in. He revised my thinking, and I know now that the inner workings of my womb will not be the focus or deciding factor when He presents me with the person he intends for me.

My friend, God is bigger than the lies the enemy tells us. We serve a God who created us and knows our worth even when we are unsure. A God who knows who we need and when we need them, and whatever He provides will not only be for our good and his glory but will be better than anything we planned and always be right on time.

WHEN WORDS PENETRATE

Our triggers are often indicators of unhealed wounds within us, highlighting areas where we need both deliverance and healing. Christian women, mainly, may experience infertility triggers differently than non-believers, as they may grapple with questions of faith, purpose, and God's plan for their lives. Spiritual triggers, such as feelings of inadequacy or guilt, can also impact Christian women, prompting us to seek solace and restoration through prayer and reliance on God's strength.

When we seek God for both deliverance and healing, we will find comfort and guidance as we navigate each challenge.

I must touch on this part briefly because it's part of my story and perhaps will be or is part of yours. Fellow believers can unintentionally trigger infertile Christian women, often through well-meaning but unhelpful comments. Statements like many women go through infertility and have children, 'Just have faith and pray and God will bless you with a child, or God has a plan for everything. These statements can inadvertently mislead and come across as dismissive. Looking back, I see how those statements were triggering to me, and perhaps what would have been more helpful would have been empathy, compassion and acknowledgement that the trial is difficult.

BE FRUITFUL & MULTIPLY

I want us to learn a lesson in being mindful of the questions we ask. Whether it's family, friends or fellow church folk, asking a woman or couple when they will have children or why they don't, may seem harmless, yet it is a very harmful question. We don't know what people are going through behind closed doors, and the habit of asking these questions needs to be addressed. When people ask this question, although unintentional, it is intrusive. I don't think people realize that long after they have walked away from the perceived harmless conversation, those of us struggling with our fertility are replaying the words for days, weeks and even years later.

While we cannot police what others say, we can control how we respond by setting boundaries regarding who we share our trial with, seeking support from understanding friends or mentors, praying for strength and guidance and asking God to equip us with the proper response when triggered. Doing so allows us to navigate such interactions with grace and resilience, fostering growth and healing in our faith journey.

I want to leave you with this not as a lesson of theology, but I pray it gives some insight into a verse often uttered. The Bible says in Genesis 1:28 ESV, "Be fruitful and multiply and fill the earth and subdue it..." When preached, the message of fruitfulness is often explained as synonymous with having children. But long before my diagnosis, when I thought of this verse, it always meant more, perhaps a foreshadowing of what would come. To be fruitful is not solely about having children. It's also about living a life that reflects the character of Christ. Fruitfulness is living a life in alignment with God to increase His Kingdom by bearing the fruits of the spirit as mentioned in Galatians 5:22-23 ESV: *"But the fruit of the spirit is love, joy, peace, patience, kindness, goodness, faithfulness, gentleness, self-control..."*

TALK IT OUT

Infertility changes how you see yourself, and through all the complexities that come along with the struggle, you have to discover your identity again in how you operate in society, but also re-establish your identity in Christ.

I want to take a moment to validate your past, present and future feelings. I understand the sense of hopelessness and fear. I understand the resentment and anger towards yourself, others and God. I understand the jealousy and sadness. I recognize the anxiety and overwhelming depression. I know the feeling of abandonment and rejection. You name it, and I understand. Every one of those feelings is valid. I also understand God's constant love and compassion for you and me. Remember, his grace and mercy are real; he has his unfailing hand in my life and yours. I want to reassure you that you are not the only one, and you do not have to do any part of this journey alone. God has not forgotten about you, nor has he abandoned you.

When a situation is a trial for one person but not another, people genuinely do not know what to say, and it's okay because it's an opportunity for you to surround yourself with praying, not prying people whose primary concern isn't the details of your situation but the healing and redemption from your situation. I encourage you to find individuals unafraid to listen to or talk about your pain no matter where you are on your journey.

I want you to be able to discern who you have in your friend and faith circles and set clear expectations. Are you seeking counsel, sympathy or a sounding board? My advice is to be clear about what you require and decide if the person in front of you can give you what you need. But before anything else, go to God and ask Him to help you and place the right people in your life during this time. If we don't talk about the pain, we can't talk about God's glory at the end of it.

**TRUST IN THE LORD
WITH ALL THINE HEART;
AND LEAN NOT UNTO
THINE OWN UNDERSTANDING.
IN ALL THY WAYS ACKNOWLEDGE HIM
AND HE SHALL DIRECT THY PATHS.**

Proverbs 3:5-6 KJV

Making crucial life decisions as a Christian can be particularly challenging due to the tensions and intertwining of spiritual considerations, personal desires and external influences.

Worldly influences often emphasize personal success, wealth, and societal approval, while Christian values prioritize spiritual growth, service to others, and obedience to God's commands. Navigating this requires discernment to ensure our decisions align with biblical principles and ultimately contribute to fulfilling God's purpose for our lives.

When facing infertility as a woman of faith, it is essential to block out the noise from well-meaning believers and non-believers alike who have an opinion on what you should do with the body God has given you but also the trial he has allowed.

Remember, God has a plan for each of us, and discerning this plan requires us to starve the outside distractions and focus on Him by developing and nurturing a deep understanding of His Word by remaining in constant communication with Him through prayer.

DISCERNMENT & DECISIONS

I was torn between the idea that waiting on God to heal me was the epitome of having faith and that proceeding with any other option outside of Him physically healing my womb meant that I lacked faith and God would be displeased with me. I didn't know what to do.

I was also plagued with the questions of the disciples in John 9: 1-2 (I'm summarizing), where they were with Jesus and came upon a man who was blind from his birth and the disciples asked Jesus *[Whose sin caused this man's blindness, was it the man or was it his parents?]* And Jesus answered and said *[it wasn't the man or his parents, but that the works of God should be made manifest in him.]*

I had the same thinking as the disciples, which left me burdened by the idea that my affliction was a direct consequence of my sins (that's where my shame came in). When that thinking is deeply rooted in your mind, healing seems inaccessible.

I was at a spiritual crossroads and understood the meaning of being between a rock and a hard place. I was stuck. I was overcome with the stress of making a decision that would affect my entire life. I was also overwhelmed that fellow Christians in my circle would deem me a person who lacked faith if I chose to have the procedure. And lastly, I was gripped by the fear of making the wrong decision overall and the idea that God would be disappointed in me. I was in a complete state of turmoil.

For many of you who are reading this and are in the same situation as I was, I offer you endless empathy. Please do not be discouraged. I ask that you surrender your body, fertility, thoughts and every part of your situation to God. I pray that you trust him enough and lay your fears, uncertainty and unbelief at his feet so He can take back his rightful place in your life. God will guide you through the decisions you need to make. Just lean in and submit to him, knowing that as He created you, He will take care of you.

TRUSTING GOD WHEN IT DOESN'T MAKE SENSE

The decision God led me to was three-fold. First, I needed to be sensitive to the spirit to hear what I was to do. Then, I needed to trust God for what He was telling me. Lastly, I needed to be obedient and do what He required.

It's interesting because we often stand on soap boxes and declare the goodness of the almighty God, but do we trust him for the things that don't make sense? I thought I did, but I struggled with the decision God led me to because it didn't make any sense. I began to waver between whether the decision was His will or mine. I wrestled with understanding how a loving God could lead me to remove the very thing I was asking him to heal—my womb.

Believing God in this decision contradicted how I thought having faith looked. Faith was believing God for your miraculous physical healing of an infirmity. The Bible demonstrated it all the time: the lame walked, the blind could see, and barren women had wombs healed that bore children. So how could I trust God when He was leading me to remove the infirmity from my body that would, by society's standards, render me incomplete and affect the rest of my life? It was removing what needed healing versus making it whole. How could I have a testimony of God's goodness and healing power if He wouldn't heal me? I questioned whether I was worth healing.

I am thankful God does not possess the limited thinking of humans. I had a limited view of how someone could receive healing; years later,

I am getting glimpses of His plan for me. What I once saw as a deficiency God has made whole in His way and timing and for his glory.

What time I am afraid I will trust in thee.
Psalm 56:3 KJV

My friend, God's will for your life may seem to contradict your plans and desires. For me, it was difficult to find peace in the journey for a very long time, but there came a point on this path when I decided to accept God's level of care and compassion for me. Through much prayer and drawing closer to God, I found peace with His will when I acknowledged his love and understood that it is against his character to steer me down the wrong path.

I gained the understanding that the decision to have a hysterectomy and tube removal wasn't a sign of a lack of faith but rather a lesson in obedience and leaning into the wisdom required for my specific situation. I don't believe living a life in constant pain and emotional turmoil was part of His plan for me, and I knew God's hand was in the decision because an overwhelming sense of peace accompanied it.

JUNE 16, 2016:
THE DAY MY LIFE OFFICIALLY CHANGED

On the day of my surgery, I was expecting that when the surgeons began my operation, they would have seen my uterus and tubes miraculously healed, and I would have the testimony of God healing my womb. My doctors and specialists would have no choice but to believe in the healing power of God and prayer and would give their lives to Christ. Wouldn't that have been something?! But it didn't happen that way. It was the opposite, as the state of my womb was worse than they thought, and that was a tough pill to swallow.

Sometimes, our healing is not a spectacular event with shock and awe; sometimes, it's the still, small voice of the Father telling us to be still and trust Him because He is by our side and is doing work on the inner parts of us that no one can see, but will manifest outwardly for His glory when he says the time is right.

My procedure lasted longer than scheduled, and the surgeon revealed the unexpected condition of my reproductive organs while I lay on the operating table. The fibroid tumours were pressing on my pelvic and spinal nerves as well as my bladder and answered the question as to why I was in so much pain in other areas of my body. To say my reproductive organs were in shambles was an understatement, and ironically, my ovaries were untouched and in perfect condition, which was a surprising sight for my surgeon and those in the room.

It's moments and information like this that remind me of the goodness of God and how he will preserve things amid a trial. God preserved and protected my ovaries as if encased in an invisible covering. The healthy state of them stopped me from needing them removed, which also stopped me from going into instant menopause. As I write this, I realize this in and of itself was and is a BUT GOD moment.

When I received my pathology report, my doctor explained that the pathologist lost count of the number of tumours and wrote that the number was inconclusive.

My gynecologist (who also performed my surgery) was consumed in tears when she visited me after surgery. She explained that she didn't realize how severe my condition was until she operated. She apologized and asked me to forgive her for making me wait so long. Little did she know God had his hand in my situation the entire time. I believe she learned and had to accept that my symptoms were not textbook, and I didn't check off the proverbial boxes on the medical diagnosis list for someone with all of the gynecological conditions I had. Unfortunately, because of this, she failed to fully believe or understand the extreme pain I had been in for nearly six years and what my body was going through daily. I hold no animosity towards my gynecologist.

My prayer for her is that when a case like mine crosses her clinic again, she remembers Talisha Matheson, the young woman whose symptoms were not textbook, who required someone to believe her and have compassion.

There were many times, as my physical body was healing after surgery, I thought perhaps I misinterpreted what God instructed me to do, but now, years later, I finally get it. How things unfolded was how God intended; I just needed to trust Him and understand that what He allowed was much bigger than my condition, the surgery and me.

THE SCARS ARE REMINDERS

I have nerve damage in my lower abdomen due to my surgeon's use of the same cut site for both surgeries. Until recently, when I touched the area, it was numb, and I barely felt my fingers on it. Today, that numbness is slowly subsiding. It's a gentle reminder that God is always working and healing, even when we least expect it. I had accepted that I would never have feeling in that area again, yet years later, He is still healing me.

The seven-inch scar across my abdomen is a reminder of the journey, and in full transparency for the longest time, I would avoid looking at it. I now realize that to ignore its existence would be to overlook the trial I went through and God's healing power. Instead of my scar being a negative reminder of my infertility, I am seeing it as a reminder of God's grace, mercy and restoration.

I want us all to be able to come to a point during our journey where we acknowledge that we may have physical, mental and emotional scars. Still, we serve a God who is the master healer and the most excellent physician we could ever ask for, and He cares for us more than we could ever ask or think.

WHY NOT THE OTHER OPTIONS?

I know many are probably wondering why I didn't navigate the other fertility options available. I wasn't going to include the reasons because it is often met with heated debate, but this book's purpose was to tell the whole story, so here I am. I had a lot of conversations with God about surrogacy, egg freezing and adoption, and my soul was never at peace for moral, ethical and spiritual reasons. And if I truly intended to follow what God had placed on my heart, I had to put other options aside and follow Him and be at peace with the outcome.

If I relied solely on logic and not spiritual, ethical or moral reasons, I chose not to freeze my eggs because it was costly, and there is a time limit on storage. I was single with no partner on the horizon, and I couldn't imagine creating a child in a lab. Egg freezing would also require a surrogate, and I couldn't imagine using another woman's womb for nine months to satisfy my desire to have a child. Surrogate offers were flooding in from well-meaning friends and family near and far, but I couldn't do it. I seriously considered adoption and researched a lot as it was the one thing I was partially open to, but I wanted the child to enter a two-parent Christian home and didn't want to adopt as a single woman.

The hysterectomy to remove my uterus and fallopian tubes significantly changed my life and my relationship with God. Physically, I felt one hundred percent better. My body was no longer fighting to stay alive and operate ordinarily, and all of the side effects I was experiencing were dwindling. My body was happy, but my soul was in an exposed state of turmoil.

SO ALSO YOU HAVE SORROW NOW, BUT I WILL SEE YOU AGAIN, AND YOUR HEARTS WILL REJOICE, AND NO ONE WILL TAKE YOUR JOY FROM YOU.

John 16:22 ESV

PROCESS OF GRIEF

Grief comes as gentle waves for some and tsunamis for others. No matter how it shows up, there needs to be an understanding for us and others that it never truly ends, no matter what type of grief you are facing, and that's okay. I want us to go through the seasons of anger, guilt, shame, and confusion; you name it, but the key is not to stay there because relief, forgiveness, restoration, and redemption are not far behind.

I believe it's important for us to know that it's okay to feel the pricks of grief years after the event that turned our lives upside down. Why? Because it's a reminder that we are still alive, and although God brought us through, he is still working on us.

PERMISSION TO GRIEVE

I didn't know grieving my fertility was required for more profound emotional healing or even if it was something I was allowed to do. I felt as if grief is and has always been reserved for those who have lost a loved one. I hadn't lost anyone, but I did lose something, and after a particularly rough session with my therapist, she gave me the permission I didn't know I needed. She told me I had the right to grieve because what I experienced was a valid loss. She explained that although I hadn't lost a child, I had lost future children and grandchildren and grieving the past, present, and future was an integral part of the healing process. So, I grieved and didn't realize how deeply it penetrated. I mourned every child I never had or will ever have. I grieved a bloodline that didn't have the opportunity to flourish beyond myself. I grieved the little girl or boy who may have looked like me and perhaps may have had dimples that matched mine. I grieved the mother and grandmother I would never be. I grieved the cousins I will never give my nieces and nephews. I grieved the grandchildren I will never give my parents and the nieces and nephews I will never give my siblings. I released myself from the guilt of everything I grieved and finally felt free.

Grief is mentally, emotionally and physically painful. There would be days when my chest would hurt, and I would feel this constraint in my throat as if I were suffocating. No two days were the same because there would be times when I was fine, with no tears and no internal pain and then days later, I would cry myself to sleep. That was when I realized grief is not linear, and I had to decide to either wrestle with it or move with it, so that's what I have done. I've moved with it. It was and sometimes still is an agonizing but necessary pain for me to accept this detour in preparation for God's lingering purpose for the rest of my life, but I am learning to continue to trust him.

I understand that grieving was necessary for me. I needed it. My soul needed it because so many people made it seem as if my infertility was and is a gift of freedom I have received. They applauded my freedom to travel and come and go as I pleased because I didn't have a family. All of that, combined with some church folk being vocal about my perceived "lack of faith" when I had my surgery, made me feel as if I didn't have a right to grieve. How wrong they were then and how wrong I was for believing it. I had every right to feel the way I felt, cry the tears I cried, and mourn every moment I mourned.

Perhaps you have been where I was or are there now, and whether you need me to say this or not, I give you permission to grieve and release everything that has you physically, emotionally and spiritually bound. I wish to hold space for you to grieve your fertility if that's where you are in your journey. I also want others in your life to hold space for you to grieve. It doesn't mean you will not emerge unharmed because there will be cuts, bruises, and many scars, but I genuinely believe it's a necessary process we must go through.

HIS DISCIPLES DID NOT UNDERSTAND THESE THINGS AT FIRST, BUT WHEN JESUS WAS GLORIFIED, THEN THEY REMEMBERED THAT THESE THINGS HAD BEEN WRITTEN ABOUT HIM AND HAD BEEN DONE TO HIM.

John 12:16 ESV

IN RETROSPECT

The modern statement that hindsight is 20/20 was proven in the Bible many times, and of course, many of us can attest to the truth as we live our lives and see God's hand (after the fact) in many of our situations. I want to preface this by stating that I would not stray from where God led me because I know the Heavenly Father divinely guided my decision. But some things were within my control that, in hindsight, I wish I had done differently, and perhaps sharing this can help arm you with a few extra tools.

PRAISE GOD IN THE VALLEY

I am fascinated by natural valleys and how they strategically run between hills and mountains. They have played a significant role in the world since the beginning of time and not only offer resources like water, healthy soils and fish, but when combined with their naturally warmer climate, they create the perfect atmosphere for growth. Winds and storms are kept at bay in the valley, and everything contained in it is naturally sheltered from the elements that could potentially harm everything within it.

Spiritually, we often view the valley as where trails take place, but I realize it is also where we are less distracted, can commune with God, and are in fellowship with him. I have learned to appreciate the valley because Jesus is the river of life and he will constantly flow through the valley with me and with you.

I will bless the LORD at all times:
His praise shall continually be in my mouth.

Psalm 34:1 KJV

LET GO & LET GOD BE GOD

I would have let God be God over my situation versus a bystander as I worried and tried everything else. Despite His knowing my thoughts and heart, I would have been consistently sincere in my approach to Him and my feelings towards him. I would have been honest with the Father because honesty is the glue that holds relationships together.

I wish I had been honest in telling him that I secretly wanted his will to match mine even after uttering, 'Not my will, Lord, but your will be done.' I wanted God to want what I wanted because I thought that would have made me content, complete and undamaged.

I have learned that once God's will is manifest, my job is to accept it as is. These days, I pray, 'Not my will but your will, Lord, please help me to be at peace, no matter the outcome.' (Some days it is easier to pray this than others, but none the less I pray it)

In letting God be God, I had to learn that whatever "thing" I was doing in God's name did not exempt me from trials or tribulations and accepting this truth pushed me into refraining from asking 'Why me?' and instead turned my inquiry into 'How are you going to use this trial for your glory?'

I understand now why God didn't use me back then. I wasn't ready to be used, and like a potter working with clay, he needed to put me back on his wheel, mould me and place me in that kiln again to refine me before he could use me and my situation.

Although I am not exactly where I thought I would be at this stage in my life because I had many plans, I am getting used to slowing down to get back into alignment with the Father, not wanting to rush ahead or lag but move in unison with him and accept exactly where he places me. We serve a glorious, magnificent and extraordinary God; knowing this, we cannot and should not limit what he can do in our lives or how he can heal us from our infirmities. I no longer want us to place God in a box and attempt to restrict His work in our lives.

THERAPY 101

I would be negligent if I didn't acknowledge that I am thankful and blessed to have a therapist who is also a follower of Jesus. This balance gives me the clinical and spiritual guidance I need, and I know only God's guiding hand strategically placed her in my life.

Therapy was something I never knew I needed until I started, and I believe God placed therapy on my heart at the right time because he saw I was ready to unpack the emotional baggage I had been carrying for so long.

To many, I looked fine on the outside, and I tried my best to maintain the façade, but in retrospect, I wasn't okay at all and should have expressed that, although in my defence, I didn't know how. I felt as if it was easier to ignore the emotional pain rather than admit to the world that the strong woman on the outside was crumbling in the depths of despair on the inside.

Now that I am armed with the knowledge of what comes with a fertility journey, I highly recommend contacting a therapist to help you maneuver through the journey—specifically, a faith-based therapist to guide you through the spiritual layer of this trial. There is something about having someone who not only has an empathetic ear to help guide you, but this person also has a relationship with Jesus.

I genuinely believe that the minute a woman is diagnosed with any form of infertility, family doctors, gynecologists and fertility specialists should have therapist recommendations on hand for their patient as well as tangible tools for those in positions of support.

Therapy is a gift. It is a chance to finally be heard, understood and supported.

— Bessel Van Der Kolk —

COMPARISON IS THE THIEF OF JOY

Comparison is something we all do or have done at some point in our lives. From the length and texture of our hair to the shape of our bodies, the clothes we wear and, yes, even the trials we face. For me, I am guilty of comparison, and something I would have done differently is not to compare my struggle and outcome with those of others, and I wouldn't have allowed anyone to impose those comparisons on me. I believe this was damaging emotionally and was challenging to overcome. People would say, '[_____] went through this, and the Lord blessed them with a child,' this is not helpful and implies that healing for infertility will result in a child and that God will heal us all the same, giving all infertile women the same testimony, which I know is not true.

When they say that comparison is the thief of joy, believe it, and I think as a Christian, comparing one person's trial and healing to that of your own takes our eyes off the one and only true Healer.

RESEARCH, RESEARCH & MORE RESEARCH

I would have researched my family history earlier to understand the heredity of my condition. During many of my doctor's appointments, I only knew a handful of relatives who had gynecological issues.
Years later, I've learned after many conversations and recalling the lives of aunts, cousins, great aunts, etc., that gynecological issues run rampant in my bloodline and that many of them struggled to have or didn't

have children not by choice, as I had assumed, but because their body wouldn't co-operate.

I wish I had known that early puberty was an indicator that something was wrong, and menstrual cramps starting at age ten were my body screaming that something just wasn't right. (As an aside, cramping associated with our menstrual cycles is not normal, and birth control, in my situation, masked a bigger life-changing problem.)

My inability to lose weight and keep it off had nothing to do with my food consumption, exercise or being lazy, as those close and not so close to me often voiced. Instead, it meant that my hormones were unbalanced and contributed to, and I believe, intensified other underlying hormonal and gynecological conditions.

The majority of the research I did resulted in contradictory information. But I will tell you what I do know about my case. Heredity played a large part in my condition. As a woman with close relatives with fibroids, I was three times more likely to develop gynecological-related issues and was medically predisposed to the condition. I still don't know or understand why fibroids specifically are mainly found in women of African descent. But one day, I hope it can be thoroughly researched and made known to us.

I encourage you to dig into your family medical history and know what ails you generationally. I believe being armed with this information will help you on your journey. For me, years after my procedure, having this information has lifted a burden I didn't know I was carrying.

MISPLACED UNDERSTANDING

To be understood is a natural human requirement for me anyway, which is why this was a massive eye-opener. Looking back, I constantly craved understanding from others regarding my situation. I was expecting empathy, but they could not give it to me. I was desiring a compassion they didn't have the capacity to provide. I missed the most critical thing during those times: God could give me everything I sought in others but on a supernatural level.

Perhaps He allowed me to be surrounded by individuals who didn't understand so I would go to Him. Eventually, I shifted my focus and kept my eyes on Him because He was and still is the only one capable of giving me what I need. Hindsight lets me chastise myself about that now because it is crystal clear. I have reconciled this with God and am using my past failure to help you, my friend.

If you are seeking all of the things mentioned above and more from your immediate surroundings, I encourage you, no, I implore you to look up because God has what you need and so much more. His word reminds us in Philippians 4:19, "But my God shall supply all your need according to his riches in glory by Christ Jesus." Our job is to trust God enough and believe Him.

JOINED A SUPPORTIVE COMMUNITY

One of my goals with this book is to set the foundation for such a space because I know I wouldn't have felt so isolated if I had a community. There would have been comfort in knowing that I wasn't the only woman who served God and was simultaneously struggling with her fertility. God created us with many emotions, and the depths of those emotions, no matter what they may be: happiness, sadness, joy, anger, you name it.

So you and I are allowed to feel all those things, and those deemed negative do not diminish our level of faith, so please, sis, feel them.

In saying this, I would have been more adamant about finding a suitable support group that aligned with my situation. Unfortunately, I joined a few online groups that were not very helpful because no one had a story similar to mine, and therefore, the understanding I was seeking was not there. Most women already had children or were well past childbearing age. There didn't appear to be space for single and infertile women, let alone within a faith-based circle, and those that I did find spun the narrative that God would heal the womb and babies would be born.

For clarification, I am not undermining God's ability to heal wombs, but I am speaking against us, believing that He will only heal a particular infirmity in a specific way. Our relationship with God is personal; therefore, our healing is individual and specific to our needs. We don't serve a cookie-cutter God, so we must avoid expecting cookie-cutter healing.

**I WILL LIFT UP
MINE EYES UNTO THE HILLS,
FROM WHENCE COMETH MY HELP.
MY HELP COMETH FROM THE LORD,
WHICH MADE HEAVEN AND EARTH.**

Psalm 121:1-2 KJV

THERE ARE LESSONS IN THE TRIAL

I asked God for healing in my body, and he gave me so much more. When I look back at where I was and the situation that I was in, I can see now that certain circumstances needed to transpire in a God-designed order.

Months before my first surgery in 2014 to remove a large fibroid tumour, God delivered me from the grips of a relationship with someone who was verbally, emotionally and financially abusing me. God gave me the courage to escape. God delivered me long before he healed me. (My God! That is an entire sermon and future conversation!) Deliverance from that situation created the foundation for me to draw closer to God in preparation for the road he knew was ahead of me. I genuinely believe had God not done what he did when he did it, I would still be in a physical and emotional state of suffering today.

RECONCILIATION WAS NECESSARY

I was at odds with God. It's a bold statement that many may not be willing to admit, but I genuinely want you to understand the depths of emotions involved. I blamed him, held him responsible for my pain, and turned my back on our relationship. I lost sight of the fact that, as my creator, he had a right to allow things to happen in my life, and I had to realize that I only inhabit this body because he decided to create me. I eventually asked God to forgive me for my feelings toward him. I had to ask him to renew my mind regarding how I viewed him and myself.

I had to reconcile and resubmit myself to Him and his will for my life, step back into alignment with him and allow him to be in his rightful place in my life.

I instigated a tug-of-war with him. I was fighting against God while he was fighting for me. And because of the sovereign God that he is, he waited for me to stop fighting and be still and approach Him in total surrender so he could finish the work he started.

I FOCUSED ON THE WRONG THINGS

I learned that I was so fixated, dare I say obsessed, with God's perceived no when it came to my fertility that I was overlooking all of the areas he was saying a resounding yes, and it took me years to recognize it. Through my pain, God was giving me a story to tell. He was equipping me with words and injecting my life with a victory that may not seem victorious to those on the outside looking in. God's perceived 'No' changed my life; perhaps the trajectory I was going on wasn't where He wanted me to be, but I am convinced this diversion was necessary to set me on the path He had intended all along.

AVOIDANCE PROLONGS SUFFERING

When friends and family had babies and baby showers for the longest time, I would find a reason not to attend the festivities. Most thought it was because I don't like forced social gatherings or large crowds, and that is true, but the real reason was that I couldn't muster up the courage to attend while feeling the way I felt about my infertility and have it not show in my facial expressions and body language. I would go through the motions of getting the gift and send it either before or after the fact, but I would never attend the showers. I couldn't bear being in spaces filled with baby bumps, infants and toddlers. My pain ran so deep that I didn't have it in me to display my happiness for them when I knew part of it was outlined in envy. There was always a reminder of what I didn't have, and those situations exposed the void in my life that I was trying to ignore.

Today, although most of my female friends are well past societal childbearing age, I don't have to contest with baby showers, infants and toddlers but rather teenage and adult humans that call me auntie, biological or not; there is joy in seeing them grow.

Baby bumps, infants and toddlers are no longer the thing that exposes a void because God did what he always does. He filled the spaces where I believed I lacked with a joy I cannot explain. It doesn't mean I never think about what could have been or the what-if of my younger years, because I do, but it does mean I am no longer consumed by it.

ADDRESSED THE ELEPHANT IN THE ROOM

I have realized the infertility conversation in most circles is taboo because of the stigma attached to the topic altogether. Speaking about infertility makes both listeners and sharers alike very uncomfortable, and I was once in that space where talking about it was far too personal and painful. In the conversation we attempt to have, listeners want to fix the perceived problem, while sharers seek safe spaces, comfort and empathy. Unfortunately, we end up being at odds, and because of this, silence fills the space where conversation, prayer and understanding should fill. There eventually comes a point on this journey when you no longer want to hide what's ailing you and realize that your pain and restoration can help someone, and even if it's one person, it's worth the risk and exposure, and our coveted privacy is no longer a factor.

I WAS HOLDING GOD HOSTAGE TO MY DESIRES

I have mentioned this before, but it's worth repeating. As hard as it may be to do, we need to give up expecting God to answer our prayers in a specific way and trust him enough to rearrange our situation according to His will and remember that he is the sovereign God who created us and knows what we need, when we need it and how we need it. I have found rest in him and no longer guard myself in his presence. Instead, I present myself as pliable and empty, so like the master potter he is, God can mould me and shape me into the vessel he intended me to be. I had to let go of the idea that God would heal me specific to my desires and trust that he would heal me. Full stop.

RESTORATION IS REAL

I had deleted something from my phone and realized days later I needed it, so I went into my recycle bin, and when I clicked on it, my phone asked if I wanted to restore it to its original folder. I said yes, and that's where it went.

We often forget the restoring power of God. He is the one who restores us, not the other way around. God is the one who brings us back to the place of redemption when we fall short. He brings us back to remembrance when the enemy reminds us of the foolish things we did in the past and wants to keep us in a place of condemnation.

The enemy will blind us with forgetfulness. He will get us to focus so much on what went wrong that we forget all of the things God has delivered us from. He will remind us of the many times we fell short then and how we fall short now. He will tell us that the Father doesn't love us because of this or that, and he uses that as a false confirmation of our supposed unworthiness when we fall. But God.

Sitting in the stillness of the Lord provides an opportunity to remember God's unfailing love and ever-stretching hand. The Holy Spirit will restore our memory with God's goodness and reveal to us the restoring power that comes with remaining close to Him and in his presence.

FOR MY SINGLE LADIES: REJECTION IS INEVITABLE

I initially removed this section and added it back at the last minute. There is no way to sugarcoat this message so I will be straightforward.
I have been rejected by men more times than I can count, solely based on my lack of fertility. At first, it stung. Actually, it was more like a punch to the jugular. There is nothing like having someone look at you as if you are a leper, as they tell you they cannot be with you because you cannot have children.

As I said at first, it's hard because the level of rejection affects you differently than if they merely said they didn't date plus-size women or women who were older or younger than them. Then you know the rejection is based on preference, and everyone has that right. But when you are rejected over something out of your biological control, it's hard to accept, and it isn't easy to not hold it against the individual. It's also hard to move past because once those words are said, they leave a scar and will inevitably affect how you show up in your next prospective relationship.

With that on the forefront of your mind, walls quickly build if you are not careful, no matter where you are on your fertility journey.
I have survived many rejections, and although I didn't escape unscathed, I have learned a few things.

First and foremost, everyone has the right to desire who and what they want in a relationship. The men who rejected me were never meant for me. Lastly, I cannot police who accepts or rejects me, but I can control how I react.

Navigating romantic relationships is hard, and if I told you single ladies that everything would be okay, it would be dishonest, and I would be doing you a disservice. Dating when you are infertile is hard. It changes who you date and how you date, and my advice is if you are not ready to openly talk about your fertility with a prospective partner in fear of him leaving, perhaps take a break from the dating scene and pray that God help you to peel back the layers and heal. Time alone and in the presence of God will allow you to come to a point where it hurts a little less, and you will eventually see rejection as redirection.

STRENGTH TO ENDURE

God doesn't give us anything we cannot handle, has become a cliché in Christian circles, especially on the lips of those who don't quite know what to say when someone is in the midst of a trial and, more specifically, to a Christian woman who is dealing with infertility. Perhaps this could be because a lot of people who say it haven't been through a similar situation or have remained tight-lipped about their struggle unless it resulted in a child.

I can honestly say that I have emerged from the ashes and that although my fertility struggle didn't result in me having a child, but rather two invasive surgeries and the scar across my abdomen as a daily reminder, my battle and yours are not wasted. It may feel like punishment, unfair, and as if there is no hope, but God created you and has prepared you, whether you feel equipped for the battle or not.

Lean into Him, sit in his presence, and allow him to work in you according to His will for your life. Relinquish where you think you should be, what you should have, who you assume you should be with, and how you believe your healing should look. Rely on who created you because He knows you better than you know yourself. God has a plan for your life and has the answers to every question, even those you have yet to ask.

Please believe me when I say there will come a point in your journey as you stick close to the Father that you will understand that the trials in our lives have been allowed to tarry because our heavenly Father wants us and others to see Him in action. So you will know that He is all-powerful, all-wise, and unconditionally loving toward you. So do not despise the difficulties. Instead, see them as a platform for God to reveal Himself to you and others.

AND WE KNOW THAT FOR THOSE WHO LOVE GOD ALL THINGS WORK TOGETHER FOR GOOD, FOR THOSE WHO ARE CALLED ACCORDING TO HIS PURPOSE.

Romans 8:28 ESV

IN MY CURRENT SEASON

*In everything give thanks: for this is the will of God
in Christ Jesus concerning you.*
1 Thessalonians 5:18 KJV

We often assume the victory over infertility is the ability to have children. It tends to be the story everyone likes to tell and the ending everyone wants because, to our simple human minds, it's the one that makes the most sense. The ending makes us the most comfortable because it satisfies our desires and gives us exactly what we want.

But what if I told you that my happy ending was a childless one and what God gave me instead was a second lease on life? He allowed this trial, which gave me the outline to tell a story of resilience, peace, hope, faith, and acceptance of a diversion that would push me to my purpose. What if I told you that my happy ending has no end and that my being here is the true answer to prayer?

I thought my healing was going to be a womb that would bear children, free from fibroids and Adenomyosis, with fallopian tubes that were not blocked. But God had a different plan in mind when it came to how He was going to heal me.

I have learned that sometimes the result of our prayers may not look how we expected them to, but it's always the way HE intended them to. It's not to say God couldn't have healed my womb because I know He can do anything. He could very well place a brand-new womb inside me today if He so chooses, but what I am saying is that although my testimony is not that of another human who can grow inside me and share my DNA, I still have a testimony.

He healed me in a way that He saw fit for the future He has planned for me. He healed me in His way for His glory. He healed my mind and my relationship with him. He healed my relationship with myself and how I viewed myself and reignited a fire in me to write and share my writing. God healed me in a way that would glorify him and help others along the way.

The revelation of my healing has been gradual. A little here, a little there. God knows me so well. He knew the best way to deal with me was to give me a little at a time so I could sit in it season after season, one revelation at a time and when it was time, he would give me the space to look back and see the whole picture.

I am living in the afterglow of God's glory and His hand on my life. It's not to say everything is perfect, but I am leaps and bounds further ahead than I was. I can openly say I no longer feel stuck, and I no longer identify with my fertility.

I am free from the bondage and the weight of expectations I put on myself and from the shame that had a hold over me. I no longer question God; instead, I am in a posture of praise and thankfulness because I am still here. I'm in my mid-forties, and I didn't expect my life to look the way it does, but I am thankful for my life and the people in it.

Sometimes, actually, most times, we want to be used by God but want it without the trial and as great as that sounds, God doesn't work that way.

I have discovered the reason for my pain and the purpose of my trial, and you are holding it in your hands or reading it on a screen right now. This book is the fruit of obedience. Obedient in going the medical route when it didn't make sense. Obedient in seeking professional counsel so long after surgery and obedient in writing a book about something so personal that I rarely had the conversation with myself, let alone put it in writing for the world to read.

I trusted God when I asked him what I should do, and I still trust him for what he has in store for the rest of my life. Reflecting on every word written, I can honestly say our God wastes nothing.

This journey was never about me. It was always about God. From before I was in my mother's womb, it was about him. When I was in her womb, and the doctors told her to abort me, God kept his hand on me and protected me for such a time as this. So, to say I know without a shadow of a doubt that I am here for a reason is an understatement.

If there is nothing else you glean from this book, I want you to know in your mind and heart that as God has created you, he will sustain you. He will never allow you to go through something you cannot bear, and even though there will be times you feel as if you just won't make it, trust his plan for your life. Trust that there is victory on the other side of the pain.

**AND HE SAID UNTO ME,
MY GRACE IS SUFFICIENT FOR THEE:
FOR MY STRENGTH
IS MADE PERFECT IN WEAKNESS.
MOST GLADLY THEREFORE WILL I
RATHER GLORY IN MY INFIRMITIES,
THAT THE POWER OF CHRIST
MAY REST UPON ME.
THEREFORE I TAKE PLEASURE
IN INFIRMITIES, IN REPROACHES,
IN NECESSITIES, IN PERSECUTIONS,
IN DISTRESSES FOR CHRIST'S SAKE:
FOR WHEN I AM WEAK,
THEN AM I STRONG.**

2 Corinthians 12:9-10 KJV

TO JOURNAL OR NOT TO JOURNAL

I am an avid journal writer, which is a significant part of my healing journey. I can honestly say journaling has saved my life and my mental health. My journal is a private space where I can let all my feelings out on paper in a judgment-free space. (There is something very cathartic about putting a pen to paper, which also gives me reasons to buy new pens and notebooks frequently.)

When I don't want to write, which doesn't happen often, I verbalize my thoughts and record everything plaguing my mind at any given time. It's never the most eloquent, but it's always a fantastic release.
Most importantly, journaling has enriched my relationship with Christ in a way I never expected, as it's been a way for me to speak to Him through written prayer. The Bible tells us, *'Do not be anxious about anything, but in everything by prayer and supplication with thanksgiving let your requests be made known to God. And the peace of God, which surpasses all understanding, will guard your hearts and your minds in Christ Jesus. Philippians 4:6-7(ESV)*

I follow Philippians 4:6-7 by writing, you can do this as well, or however you choose to communicate with God. The most important thing is that you remain in communication with Him even when you feel you have nothing to say because the Holy Spirit can and will speak to you in your moments of stillness and silence.

I have provided several questions that can serve as journal prompts that may help you as you continue journaling or begin the habit. Please be honest because I don't want you to write what sounds good. I want you to be honest with yourself and God because that is where we all find freedom.

My friend, I pray these questions will help you move through your journey as much as they helped me.

1. How am I feeling right now? Be Honest
2. What do I need to release? What is keeping me stuck?
3. If I could talk to someone about where I am in my journey, what would I want them to know?
4. What is something I want my partner to know during our fertility journey?
5. What do I want people to stop saying to me concerning my infertility? Why? How can I articulate this to them?
6. How can my partner help me during our fertility journey? How can I help him?
7. What boundaries do I need to set during this time that will aid in my healing and throughout this journey?
8. What are my fertility triggers?
9. What are healthy ways I can manage my triggers?
10. What brings me joy that is non-fertility related?
11. Does my fertility consume me? How am I consumed? Why am I consumed?
12. What positive steps can I take to reduce being consumed by my fertility?
13. What feelings surface when I think about my fertility?
14. How do I view God concerning my fertility?
15. If my body could talk, what would it say?
16. How has my relationship with God changed during my fertility journey?

17. What does God's word say about who He is and who I am to him?
18. What was my relationship with God like before I knew about my infertility? What is it like now?
19. What am I grateful for at this moment?
20. List the questions you need answers to, and write who can provide that answer beside each one.
21. When my journey gets tough, what is something I want to remember?
22. Write an honest letter to God and tell Him exactly how you feel at this particular moment.
23. What is God telling me to do vs what I want to do? Be honest.
24. Find a Bible verse to meditate on for the next month.
25. Am I isolating myself or surrounding myself with others? Explain why.
26. List your doubts and how God can turn doubts into hope.
27. Am I in alignment with God? What do I need to do to draw closer to God? Be honest.
28. Have I submitted my fertility and my situation to God? Why or why not? Be honest.
29. Why do you believe you are in this trial? Be honest, What does the Bible say about it?

A FINAL WORD OF ENCOURAGEMENT

It isn't in burying your feelings that you find meaning and triumph-it's in taking them to Him.

– unknown -

Friend, as we end this book, I pray you have found hope among these pages. I want to encourage you that even when you don't know how things will turn out, God will give you comfort, hope, and a peace that transcends your understanding.

I genuinely believe that when God allows difficulties in our lives, He will bring forth some good purpose from them. So don't imagine that the trials and delays you're experiencing are because of the Father's contempt for you. Instead, know this is the perfect platform to witness His glorious intervention on your behalf.

As you walk through your fertility journey, remember that your worth and identity are not defined by your ability to conceive because, above that, you are a beloved child of God. Although your journey will be filled with challenges and uncertainties, trust in the Lord's plan for your life, for He promises to give you hope and a future. As you move forward, may you find strength in your faith, courage in your resilience, and comfort in knowing you are never alone. Your story is still unfolding, with God by your side, no matter where you are on the journey. Every chapter holds the promise of miracles yet to come. Keep believing, hoping, and shining your light for His Glory. Remember, when Jesus steps on the scene, change is inevitable.

My prayer is that you go to Jesus and tell him that you need his help to make sense of all that has happened and is happening. Ask him to give you his comfort, hope and peace as you process it.

May God Bless & Keep You.

PRAYER

Eternal God and Father, we thank you for the air in our lungs, the beating of our hearts and the freedom to serve and communicate directly with you. Father, I Thank You for allowing the trial and for allowing me to emerge from the ashes because I know it was all for your glory, and you wasted nothing. From the moment you said yes to me in my mother's womb to this moment as I type these final words, you have had your hand on me, and for that, I am thankful.

Father, I pray for every woman holding this book and ask that you cover her from the top of her head to the soles of her feet and provide her with the comfort she needs during this time.

Father, I ask that you surround her so she never feels alone or abandoned. I ask that you wipe every tear that falls from her eyes and cancel out every feeling of guilt, shame and defeat. I ask that you renew her mind of any angst and confusion. I ask that you remove the scales from her eyes and help her to see herself as you see her.

Lord, I pray for the souls reading this who do not know you and that you soften their hearts, and they will come to know you and enter into a relationship with you.

Father, we thank you for what you have done, what you are doing and in advance for what you will do in every one of these lives. Lord, we give you all the honour, all the praise and all the glory in Jesus' mighty name.
Amen!

**BEAR ONE
ANOTHER'S BURDENS,
AND SO FULFILL
THE LAW OF CHRIST.**

Galatians 6:2 KJV

JOIN THE COMMUNITY!

We all need a safe place to land no matter where we are in our fertility journey, and beyond popular belief, this place can reside outside of our circle of lifelong friends and family. That is where the **Sisterhood of Faith & Hope** comes in. We are a community of God-fearing women in different stages of our fertility journey. We have created a God-centered space where we will discuss, encourage, support, rejoice and pray one another through the hilltop and valley moments in this life-impacting journey. It will be an edifying and fruitful experience.

If this sounds like the community for you, join us by emailing **info@theinspiredintrovert.com** or by following and messaging me on IG **@theinspiredintrovert_**

BE INSPIRED!

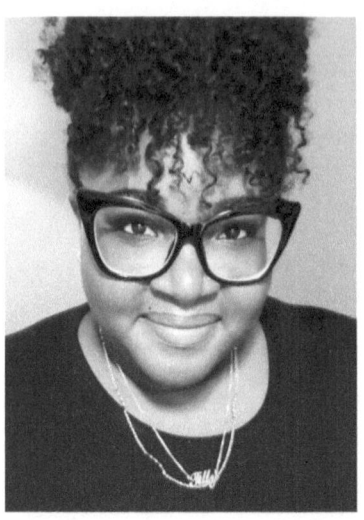

Also, by Talisha A Matheson

The Little Book of Introverted Thoughts – Vol 3
The Little Book of Introverted Thoughts – Vol 2
The Little Book of Introverted Thoughts
Soul Talks: 52-Weeks of Inspiration

Email: info@theinspiredintrovert.com
Web: www.theinspiredintrovert.com
Instagram:@theinspiredintrovert_